SKINNY BAD BITCHES

& What THEY DO TO GET & STAY THAT WAY

ALSO BY SHERRIMA QUEEN:

Dragonflies in Hollywood: Everything That Shines Ain't No Diamond

@ Amazon.com & Barnes & Noble

Cover design: Khaila Batts

Drawings : Creative Illustrations Studio

This book has been cataloged as a self-help, weight loss, lifestyle, nonfiction.

This book is dedicated to all my Bitches = Queens committed to a healthy lifestyle.

Forward

I'm going to start off by saying that all women's body shapes are beautiful. It doesn't matter if you're fat, skinny or somewhere in between. It's important to embrace your body in the size you are RIGHT NOW because YOU ONLY GET ONE. So enjoy every stage of your womanhood. In addition, when you accept yourself the way you are, you subconsciously give others permission to accept you too.

On the other hand, if there's something you don't like about your body, you have the power to change it. You don't need a lot of money, but I would be lying if I said money doesn't speed up the process. For example, you can go the surgery route, but this instant gratification won't teach you lifestyle changes and there's a big chance your body will revert back to its former fat self. You can also hire a personal trainer. Exercise is good whether you're being coached or doing it on your own, but once again, if you don't change your eating habits and learn what's best for your body, you'll find you've wasted your money. However, if a bitch doesn't have enough cash or has limited credit, she has to go to Plan B, which should really be Plan A: Relearning how to eat.

This book is your Plan B.

If you follow the program described in this book, you will be amazed at how fast you will reach your goals. If, when you look in the mirror, you repeat to yourself a zillion times, "I love my body" but still hate it, Bitch, this book is for you!

If you read Cosmopolitan, Marie Claire or Essence and fantasize about being the size of the women in those magazines, this book is for you, too. You can never change your body *type*, but you can make your type the best it can be.

So what do Rihanna, Kim K, J.L0, and Madonna have in common besides being in the entertainment business? I'll tell you. They all have a small waist and they're skinny, curvy BAD BITCHES who slay. So can you! Yeah, they're rich and famous, but you can get a body like theirs from following the program in this book.

This book is for any woman who wants to lose weight or maintain a "Skinny Bad Bitch" body, which I will refer to as "SBB." And it doesn't matter how old you are. By following this program, you will be incorporating a more nutritious and conscious lifestyle. It's not about being vain. It's about being the best version of you in this lifetime and it's never too late. If you're reading this book, either you're already a SBB or one lies somewhere inside you and she's ready to come out, dammit. This book is for all women, and even men! Yes, sweetie men can be Skinny Bad Bitches too!

In this book, I share diet and lifestyle secrets that a SBB won't tell you, but I will. I have been around SBBs my entire life and I've studied nutrition and holistic food. I know the power of food and how it can transform you. Many women have come to me for advice and guidance and this is the main reason I wrote this book. I believe everyone should have access to this information.

In addition, I have changed my own body in the process and I want to share my knowledge with you.

I purposely made this book a short easy read without all the long medical terms, complicated jargon and pain-in-the-ass calorie counting. The modern woman is on the go. She's career oriented: Mommies, wives, students, bosses - basically just hard working - who don't have time to waste. Health is number 1 for the modern woman. That's why I briefly explain why you should stay away from certain foods that can cause weight gain and possibly lead to disease. One great thing about this program is that you don't have to deny yourself all the foods you love. It's all about:

- ❖ Moderation for some of the foods you love that might not be that good for you
- ❖ Taking away the really bad stuff completely
- ❖ Adding other foods that will work hard to edify your body so it can do what it's supposed to do

I encourage you to take from this book what feels right for you. After all, you have free will; just remember that to continue taking the same actions and expecting a different result is the definition of insanity.

So jump right in, digest the material (no pun intended), make the lifestyle changes, reach your goal, and slay. It's that simple!

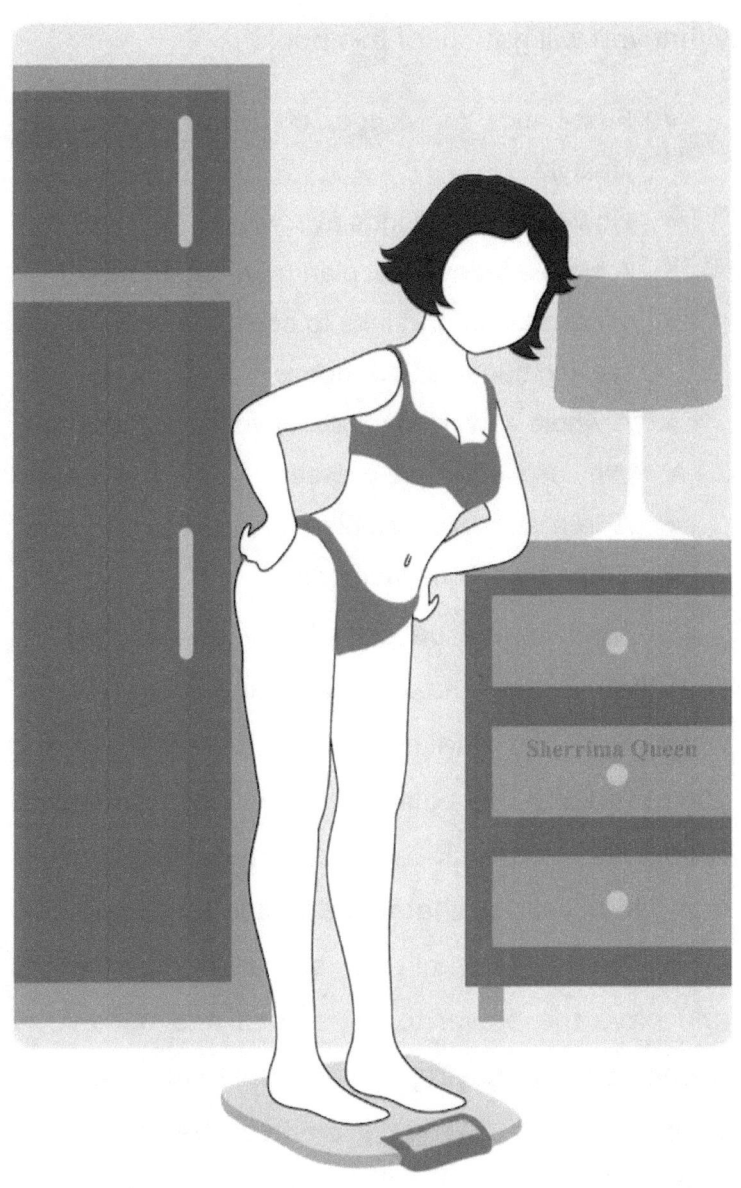

What you will get out of this book:

- First-hand knowledge of SBB secrets and lifestyle
- How to lose 5 pounds every week
- A simple 5-day meal plan (non-complicated)
- What snacks or drinks to consume when you're craving sugar, salt or booze
- A whole new mindset about your body and spirit
- Why as women we overeat
- A "realistic" exercise plan
- Some humorous moments

Now I must be completely candid and tell you that it does take *vision* and *commitment*, which are two qualities all SBBs have, and if you're reading this book, you have it too. However, if you feel you lack these qualities, this book is going to show you that you do have them and how to use them. After all, we are all human beings and have the power to set a goal and achieve it. Remember the saying "Fake it until you make it"? Well, I like to say "Think it until you believe it" and that's what you'll do. So if you're ready to get started on your SBB journey, continue reading!

Table of Contents

Chapter 1.

THE REASONS WE MISTREAT OUR BEST FRIEND FOREVER (BFF)

Weight loss is about the relationship you have with your body. Your body is your best friend forever. If you're good to her she will take care of you. That's why it's important to say loving affirmations to your body and feed it the proper fuel. Even if you're not at your desired weight yet. Yes, tell your body every day that you "love it" when you look in the mirror.

Most overweight people are overweight for three reasons. Either they're trying to protect themselves, they're emotional eaters, or they just don't give a shit.

The Protective Eater

A lot of women eat unconsciously and there are any number of psychological reasons for this.

One of them, believe it or not, is to get fat. The extra weight becomes a shield. It's a way for people to leave them alone, or not consider them a threat. For example, how many women have you seen with beautiful faces that were fat? You look at them and say to yourself, "if she lost weight she would be so pretty." I'm sure many! I interviewed some of these women for this book and all of them told me that they were molested when they were a child. I'm not saying all women that are fat or overweight were molested but the ones I talked to were.   They used the extra weight to keep men from noticing them sexually. Once I mentioned that reasoning some of them said that they had never thought of it that way.

The Emotional Eater

Now, the emotional eater overeats to change her mood. I'm guilty of that one, big time. Think about it, if you're depressed or something is worrying you, you go for a snack. It's tempting to grab for something that's going to stimulate the senses immediately and take your mind off whatever it is you may be anxious about. So you reach for something yummy, comfort food; for example a piece of chocolate cake with vanilla ice cream. You immediately get a jolt of happiness and it changes your mood. Then after that it's just a matter of time before that feeling fades and you're depressed again looking for your next fix. I know the feeling all too well. Just to let you know, many researchers have found sugar to be highly addictive equivalent to a drug. So it's not really our fault. I'll explain more a bit later about the addictive nature of sugar and what happens to your brain when you eat it.

The Don't Give A Shit Eater or Hormones

The painful reality is that after a certain age or after having a baby, some women lose their discipline or suffer from postpartum depression caused by a severe hormonal imbalance.

Post-partum depression occurs when hormone levels rise in a woman who's pregnant. After the baby is born, hormone levels suddenly drop causing the depression. Sometimes this causes women to overeat and become overweight or fat. Some women develop the mindset that they can't lose weight therefore they become depressed and don't try. By the way this condition is treatable.

I have met women who stop watching what they eat and exercising after they turn 35. Then again some women were never taught proper nutrition so they might not know what a balanced healthy meal is. I'm not judging but I feel once you reach a certain age it's your responsibility to seek information that will help you evolve as a person. Then again you have to desire it and take action.

If you're still eating the same junk food you ate as a teenager and you're 35 or 50 years young, something is wrong. It's likely you're going to get fat because your metabolism has changed. Not to be negative but after 40 years of age most people become comfortable with their size because they believe they're old now. Not everyone, but a large percentage of people think that way. Which in my opinion is ridiculous.

Unfortunately, some people don't try to get rid of the weight they've gained.

I've heard women make comments like, "Girl, I got my husband or my man so I'm off the market." Basically, they stop giving a shit because they have their spouse. Then when their husband starts creeping, they get mad at the side chicks, calling them homewreckers. What I have learned is that women are quick to jump at each other because it's easier to blame the woman as opposed to the person you actually have the relationship with. I blame men for this kind of behavior.

When I was 27 years old I went to Los Angeles. In Starbucks I met this older man, I guess he had to be about 55 then. The man and I started talking and he asked me my age. I told him I was 27 years old. I will never forget this; he told me that I was old, but said it in a nice way. I looked at him bewildered. I'm old? I wasn't the same person I am today so I didn't respond and merely camouflaged my hurt. The comment made me feel very insecure. Can you believe the irony of that coming from a man close to 30 years older than I was?

Some men purposely try to create insecurities in women to control them. Unfortunately, this has been going on for centuries and it's one of the main reasons women have to develop a strong sense of self - so ignorant comments like that won't affect you. My point in telling this story is that I want you to know I understand why some women feel once they have their spouse or husband, they can let themselves go because they got the prize: a man.

So how do you get past negative comments, see-sawing hormones, childhood or teen traumas, and current emotions? In other words, how do you begin to give a shit again about taking control of your weight and your health?

Know what you want, take action and keep it sexy.

A SBB has many life goals. For example, one could be career related, so she strategizes on how to get that promotion or how to start that business. Similarly, in this book, we're going to strategize on how to love your body, get it where you want it and keep it that way.

My goal in this book is to have you a Skinny Bad Bitch with a little fat in the right areas, so we're going to set a plan of action.

But first, let's take a look at that 5/6 of the brain that's doing all your thinking for you to see how it works and why, including why thinking yourself thin should be part of the plan. This is where the magic is going to happen.

Chapter 2.

Your Brain Believes What it Thinks You Want it to Believe

By default, you are currently a victim of your environment, your upbringing and your experiences. Everything you know – or think you know – has shaped who you are. The product known as you is the brainchild of the world in which you live.

What you believe about yourself and your world is a mirror reflection of everything you've learned, whether it was through the natural world, by educators or parents or by encountering others. By understanding the evolution of thought, you'll begin to see how your thoughts can work against you or for you. The choice has always been yours.

How you think is as important as what you think about. Your brain will always default back to what it knows. In other words, if you've been fat for a while and that's how you see yourself, you need to re-imprint your brain with thoughts that tell it you're skinny. And you need to phrase it in a positive way. Don't say "I'm not fat" or "I can beat this fatness" or "Fat will no longer control me". Instead say, "I'm skinny", "I'm healthy and whole and beautiful", "My body has found its perfect balance and shape" or something similarly positive.

Your brain doesn't know the difference between thought and reality, between experience and virtual experience. It only remembers the way something made you feel. So emotions are a huge component in this equation. Each time you recite a positive mantra, believe it to be true, feel it, visualize it in your mind; see yourself as a skinny bad bitch moving around your kitchen preparing healthy foods grooving to the music, wearing a svelte dress or sashaying down the runway. Any image you create is the right one, but you must *feel* it.

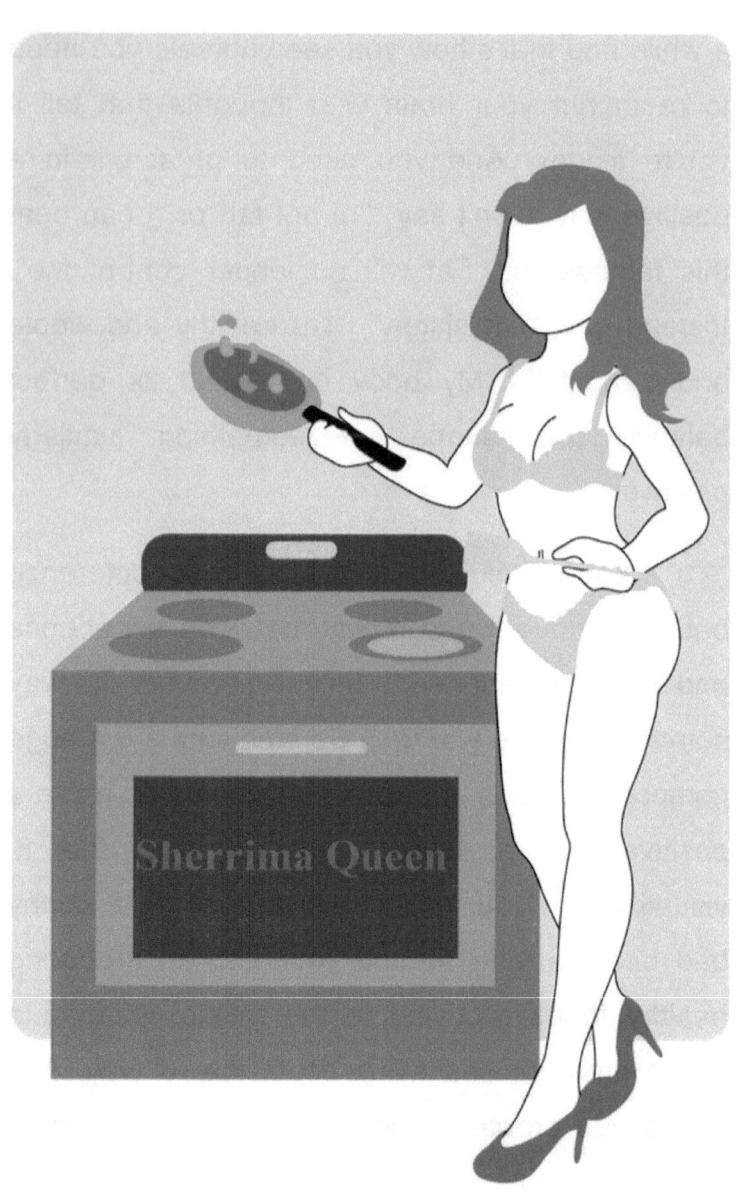

Chapter 3.

How Food Works

Some people confuse fat with curvy. I know some men love women with big butts, and it does look sexy, but you have to have that waist snatched—translation: you need to get it small.

In order to lose weight, you have to be particular about what you put in your mouth, plain and simple. You have to become a food snob. First of all, just like a good makeup artist knows the importance of using the right products, shades and manipulation to get the look she wants, a SBB knows the importance of diet – how food works and which foods work best for her.

Now, when I say diet, I'm not talking about eating rabbit food or bingeing on diet sodas that may lead to cancer. (Let's not forget about how some women walk around with a bad attitude because they're hungry and starving themselves to stay skinny). I'm talking about eating food that not only tastes good, but also fills you up and gives your body what it needs. Food should nourish the body and give you energy, and as a result, you glow. Last, but not least, it puts you in a positive state of mind because your mind, body and spirit are aligned, so you're always on fleek.

Foods that taste good but you know are not good for you need to be either at a minimum in your diet or eliminated altogether. You have to trick your brain into thinking that these foods will make you sick, literally. And this goes back to imprinting the brain with what it thinks is real. For example, fatty foods or desserts high in empty calories. When you're tempted, tell your mind, "if I eat this it will make me sick". "I might possibly vomit", and eventually that's exactly what will happen. Give yourself about 2 months. Believe me, you won't desire it anymore.

So What's Up With Sugar?

I told you I would explain more about the addictive nature of sugar and what happens to your brain when you eat it.

It might be interesting for you to realize that you can and probably have become tired of eating real whole food at some point, maybe often. You try to eat right, but you just get bored with it. So why is it that you never get sick of ice cream, cake or other sweets? What is it about sugar that's so addicting?

Sugar is a carbohydrate that increases dopamine, a neurotransmitter that spikes whenever we do something pleasurable (like eating ice cream or having sex). This in turn sends a signal to the part of your brain that asks "was this a pleasurable experience?" Yes, it was. You know this consciously and your brain knows it subconsciously, so you eat more sweets. But what begins to happen is that your tolerance for sugar increases so your brain is never satisfied. It always wants more, just like a drug. This leads to cravings, weight gain, unregulated blood sugar which can lead to diabetes, imbalances that affects the skin, hair, cognition, mood, perception, and a host of other ailments.

Tricking your brain will take some time, but it can be done. It's a matter of science, not will. And it begins with setting your goal.

How Much Weight Do You Want To Lose?

Determine a healthy weight based on your body type and size and make sure you write it down. Writing it down in a diary or food journal will activate your subconscious mind to help you accomplish your goal faster. Set a small goal first like 10 pounds in two months. I don't want you to put too much pressure on yourself too soon, and get frustrated and quit. On the other hand, if you're ambitious you can set your goal for a shorter period of time. To be candid, that's how I lost 10 pounds in one month and kept it off. I weighed all my portions with my food scale that you can purchase from SkinnyBadBitches.com. It's great! In addition, I became a vegetarian. I had lost my desire for eating meat. I was obsessed with changing my lifestyle, but the choice ultimately is up to you.

Write the size you want to be on a few sticky notes and place them on your refrigerator, mirror and one in your purse. I know it might sound weird, but it works because it reminds you of your goal. I even put a sticky note on my cell phone case.

Next, imagine in your mind the size you want to be. If you can't visualize it, get a picture of someone who is the size you want to be and hang it on your refrigerator. I used to have a picture Janet Jackson. I always loved her body because she was skinny but strong and muscular. I always loved dancers' bodies. To me they have the best bodies in the world. The picture you choose will be your motivation.

The more you're reminded of your goal, the more you will think about it and do what's necessary to achieve it. That's just how the brain works.

Chapter 4.

MEAT OR NOT TO MEAT? THAT IS THE QUESTION

It has been proven that people who eliminate meat from their diet lose weight faster. However, for the purpose of this book, I'm going to assume you like a little meat every now and then. I have to tell you though, a SBB who does eat red meat minimizes the quantity she consumes. Most SBB's usually keep it to no more than once a week. They won't tell you that, though!

Just for the record, though, I have to say that eliminating meat from your diet is healthier for you. Omitting red meat keeps a high percentage of fats from entering the body. When you eat red meat, it takes 72 hours or more for your body to digest it, so it sits in your intestines for days before it comes out the other end. Really, who wants to be full of crap for several days? And combining meat with starches or carbohydrates in one meal (like meat and potatoes, pasta and meatballs, hamburger on a bun) causes you to feel bloated and your stomach to protrude. To make matters even worse, you start to feel tired or sluggish. A SBB has no time for that. They have places to go and people to see!

I also have to inform you about all the crap that's being injected into animals these days which we turn around and put into our bodies.

Conventional animals are raised in large CAFOs (Confined Animal Feeding Operations) where they're over-crowded, live in their own feces, eat through iron fences, are fed GMO grains (cows are not designed to eat grains), are given hormones to fatten them quickly, and are routinely given antibiotics so they don't get sick. They're also not removed from the herd when they do get sick. This practice is causing an increased resistance to antibiotics among humans.

If you really love meat, stick to grass-fed animals. They're no more pricy than other meat if you purchase them directly from a farm. Go online to find a farm near you where you can pick up meat produced from healthy, pastured animals.

USDA certified organic beef is the next best thing to pastured beef. Organic principles don't allow GMOs in feed, but cows are still fed grains. They're also not given antibiotics, hormones or steroids. Organically raised and pastured cows rarely get sick, but when they do, they're removed from the herd and not replaced even when they return to health.

OMG, I'm surprised that, given all the stuff they're injecting into cows and pigs now, we humans haven't turned into mutants yet. So please be selective when choosing to eat red meat.

Now, if you can't get away from the meat right away or you don't have a desire to, it's OK, I get it. I know meat is tasty; I did indulge at one time in my life. I'm aware that most restaurants don't serve USDA certified organic beef. The next alternative would be 100% Angus beef, however, definitely stay away from pork. I know some of you are reading this and saying is this bitch crazy? I need my bacon!! Don't put pork on your fork if you want to be a Skinny Bad Bitch. An alternative to pork bacon is turkey bacon. Turkey bacon has less fat and calories but it contains a lot of sodium. The reason pork is not good for you is because of the pig's diet, and unfortunately they don't have organic pig.

I mentioned vegetarian because this lifestyle has become popular in our society. New York City, for example, has so many awesome vegetarian restaurants and the food is delicious. Trader Joe's and Whole Foods are two supermarkets that many vegetarians shop at. If you decide to become a vegetarian or vegan, it is a great option for weight control. However, most people do it because of the cruelty to animals. I'm not trying to convert anyone into becoming a vegetarian. I'm only reminding you of the options you have.

HOW A SBB DINES OUT

You're out with friends and everyone at the table orders a cheeseburger, medium rare, with fries. Unapologetically, you, the Skinny Bad Bitch orders a burger (100% beef) no cheese, lite cheese or if the place is bougie, goat cheese on whole grain bread or bun. If you're a vegetarian, you order a veggie burger with mozzarella or vegan cheese. Instead of ordering fries, you, the SBB, orders a salad with dressing on the side, so you can control the amount you use. (Some dressings are filled with high amounts of sugar, sodium, fat, and artificial ingredients your body doesn't recognize as food, and these ingredients put weight on the body. This is why I strongly suggest salad dressings that are vinegar and olive oil based. For example, balsamic vinaigrette or lite Italian.)

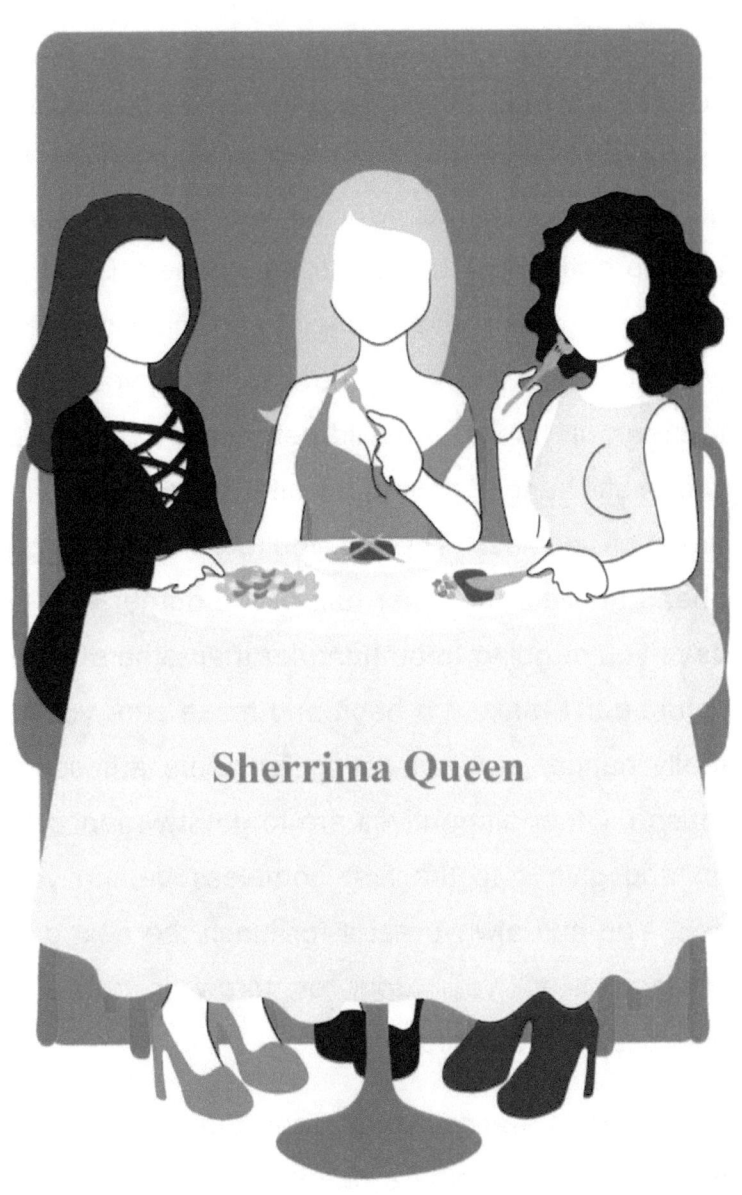

Sherrima Queen

Back to dining: You're a Skinny Bad Bitch so only eat half of the burger. Have the waiter immediately wrap the other half of your burger to go because if you leave it on your plate you will end up eating it. Trust me. I have done this many times and I wasn't even hungry. I believe it's called a habit. That's why every now and then you have to break up habits. I would bet money on that! If you're still hungry, have the waiter bring you a side order of veggies. Then, if you're still hungry, go ahead and eat the other half of the burger. Some days you're going to be hungrier than others, I get it; just don't make it a habit and make sure you're really hungry and not eating for some emotional reason. Other alternatives are to get it wrapped to go and give it to the first homeless person you see. You can always eat it for lunch the next day or feed it to your dog, or throw it out, not necessarily in that order.

When eating steak, eat the leanest cut possible; top sirloin is a good choice if they don't carry USDA organic beef. It has less than 5 grams of total fat. I know top sirloin steak is a little pricey, but like L'Oreal says, you're worth it. What's the point? Toxins are stored in the fat of animals, humans included. So when you eat the fat, you're getting all the pesticides, fungicides, herbicides, steroids, and antibiotics that were given to the animal in a concentrated form.

Chapter 5.

NO COUNTING CALORIES: IT'S ABOUT PORTION CONTROL AND EATING REAL FOOD

Most SBBs aren't into counting calories. It's too time consuming and confusing. Who really has time to be adding up numbers every time they eat? On the other hand, I am a strong believer in portion control. The United States Food and Drug Administration (FDA) states, in order to have a well-balanced diet, you need to eat from the following food groups daily: fruits, vegetables, proteins, grains.

The new federal guidelines say fruits and vegetables should consume half of the food on your plate. I believe vegetables should consume your plate more than fruit but try both ways and see what's best for your body.

The best guide for portion control is your hand when you're dining out however when you're home use a food scale for more accuracy. You can purchase our food scale on our blog. It's designed especially for SBB's. When using your hand it's relatively simple. To measure your consumption:

- ❖ Take your hands and ball up two fists; put them together and that is the amount of fruit you should eat daily or have on your plate. If it's whole fruit like an apple or banana that's equivalent to half the plate fruit requirement.
- ❖ Put two fists together again and that would represent the amount of veggies you should have on your plate.
- ❖ The amount of protein that is suggested is 7 ounces, which is approximately the size of one fist. I must say, the amount of protein needed for your body depends on your age and level of physical activity. However 7 ounces is about average.
- ❖ As far as whole grains, we are looking at 6

to 7 ounces, which is also about the size of 1 fist.

❖ Add to that small amounts of dairy and healthy fats.

Now a SBB keeps dairy to a minimum. For example, you can put milk in your coffee or cereal, try to choose organic almond, soy or rice milk, particularly, soy should be organically grown and whole because of the naturally occurring phytoestrogens that can affect hormones. They're healthier for you, once again, because of the chemicals being injected in cows. So if you have to drink milk, don't drink more than 3 ounces a day and make sure it's fat free or organic.

Goat milk is an excellent alternative to cow milk. It has the same type of taste, but is milder. Goats are not raised in CAFOs and have far less naturally occurring fat and estrogen in their bodies.

Healthy fats include coconut, olive, walnut, and avocado oils. Make sure they're cold-pressed and ethically processed. Avocados, nuts, almond or cashew butter, sunflower seeds, and coconut meat or cream are good vegetarian sources of fat. Eggs are another healthy source of fat provided they're from free-range or organically raised chickens.

In addition to portion control, watch your sugar and salt intake. They are also culprits of weight gain. If you're used to eating processed and packaged food, learn to read labels. Don't eat more than 450 mg of sodium and 30g of sugar in a single day. Eventually, however, you will learn to do away with processed and packaged foods altogether as they generally lack nutrients.

CHAPTER 6.

ARE YOU A CHICKEN OR JIVE TURKEY?

Yes, even a SBB has a few moments of weakness, but those moments don't outweigh her overall vision, which is to stay or become a SKINNY BAD BITCH!

Every morning a SBB imagines herself on the scale weighing their dream weight through meditation. A SBB is neither a chicken nor a Jive turkey. She eats them for lunch or dinner, preferably grilled in her salads or sautéed in whole-wheat penne pasta. By the way a SBB never eats fried chicken, or keeps it to a minimum. I know some of you are probably reading this and saying, "Okay, you're having another crazy moment, bitch, right!"

Fried chicken -- I know, it's so good. Even right now my mouth is watering just thinking about it, but it's so bad for you! Now, I know even a SBB has moments of fuck it. If you get one of those moments and have to have that fried chicken, DON'T EAT THE SKIN! I know you're saying, "But the skin is the best part." Just to let you know, the skin of fried chicken is equivalent to that booty call that comes over at midnight and gives it to you real good. The only thing is, after it's all over, he or she wants to borrow $100 that you know darn well you ain't getting back.

Basically, what I'm saying is, there is a price you're going to pay for eating the skin, so just be prepared to pay it, not only on your waistline but also on your complexion. Too much grease clogs your pores and your arteries, which can lead to a heart attack. Eat your chicken grilled, baked, sautéed or boiled. However, if you're going through that fuck it moment, don't exceed fried food more than once a week. Seven ounces is two average pieces of chicken. For example, a wing and a leg (a Number 2 at Kentucky Fried Chicken).

Side note: the long-term goal is not to eat fried food at all. Once you refrain from it, your body will no longer crave it. It takes 28 to 60 days to break a habit. Remember that!

You may not be a jive turkey but you definitely love to eat them, unless you're vegetarian. Which, by the way, would be the highest dietary goal for a SBB. Eliminating meat puts your energy on a certain universal frequency; however, that's another book. Back to the subject at hand, turkey is lean, rarely fried and it tastes good. A turkey sandwich with light or vegan mayo, avocado and a kale salad on the side would be the perfect SBB lunch.

After the first week of following the regimen in this book, you will have more energy, feel lighter and see yourself getting slimmer. In addition, your personality may change. Some may describe it as feeling "airheadish". The reason for this is because your body is purging old crap including toxins and waste from flushing fat.

I have created a 5-day meal plan for you to

follow. You can substitute foods and again I stress portion control. On the other hand, I highly suggest sticking to the program in this book if you want to see results faster. I will give you a list of suggested foods. Once the weight starts falling off, which it will, you will be excited because you're becoming the person you really want to be. It's also important to keep a positive attitude. Some people may find it challenging the first couple of weeks, but push through it, SBB. You will reach your goal.

Chapter 7.

SOUP AND SALADS

SBBs eat salads and soups as often as possible, not because they follow stereotypes but because of the nutritional value. Soups and salads are light and taste good, and you can always add whole grains to the mix if you're still hungry, like bread. Yes, I said bread!

Most guys say they like a woman who loves to eat. They claim that they don't want a salad-eating woman, but those are the ones they marry. Where do you think the term "trophy wife" came from? I personally don't see anything wrong with being a trophy wife, as long as each person gets what he or she wants from the relationship, but that's another book too. So, girl, eat your salads.

❖ Add as many vegetables as possible. I guarantee, after that, he's going to want to toss your salad.

❖ Don't forget to eat small amounts of protein

at every meal. If a SBB is really hungry, they usually add chicken, turkey or seafood to their salads, but you can add nuts, seeds or quinoa.

❖ Add a small amount of healthy fat either in a dressing or by adding nuts, avocados, or seeds.

❖

Spinach, kale and mix green lettuces are the favorite greens of SBBs. I recently caught several SBBs eating some Chinese lettuces called bok choy and Shanghai bok choy. I asked them, what is that? At first, they hesitated to tell me and I said, "Bitch you better spill the tea. I'm writing a book." So, one of them told me and let me try it. OMG, it was so good. Both lettuces were flavorful and filled with nutrients. You can get them mostly from Asian markets. In addition, greens contain flavonoids, antioxidants that work to detoxify the body. Greens also keep the skin soft and the complexion smooth.

Soups are another great way to get your veggies, protein and fat all in one meal. Here are a list of Low sodium, awesome soups to indulge in include:

- ❖ Tomato basil
- ❖ Carrot
- ❖ Lentil
- ❖ Chicken noodle
- ❖ Black bean
- ❖ Broccoli
- ❖ Miso
- ❖ Vegetable

It's always best to make your own so you can control the ingredients, but if you read labels, you can enjoy packaged or canned soups from the supermarket..

Chapter 8.

CRAVING SWEETS

Whenever a SBB has a sugar craving, especially around that time of the month or when feeling a little melancholy, she knows what to do to lift her spirits. She eats fruit, drinks one glass of wine or has a small piece of dessert. After that, she goes and looks at the photo on her refrigerator for strength and says "God help me". Then focuses her mind on her desired weight.

However, if you're having a serious sugar craving like a crackhead on crack, dark chocolate is your fix! Dark chocolate is considered a superfood, therefore it has nutritional value. What is a superfood? It's a nutrient-rich food considered to be especially beneficial for health and well-being. Dark chocolate is made from the cocoa tree. It has soluble fiber and is loaded with minerals. Dark chocolate is also an aphrodisiac; I can attest to that!

When eating dessert, it's all about portion control. That's why a SBB monitors her sugar intake. White refined sugar is a killer on the body in more ways than one. Not only does it cause weight gain, but too much sugar has also been linked to diabetes and cancer. I know these days everything contains sugar, so that's why a SBB reads ingredients. Therefore, when eating dessert, don't eat more than 2 ounces, which is about the size of your thumb.

A SBB at a Party: you're at a birthday party and they're passing out cake. You, a SBB, graciously accepts a slice to be polite, even though you don't really want it, I think. You then take a tiny piece of the cake, I'm talking the size of a string bean. When no one is looking, you, a SBB pretend to take another bite, but instead you discreetly mash the cake with your fork while having a conversation with others. No one notices anything. Then say, "OMG, this cake is so good" and throw it out! I personally have witnessed this and done this myself. It works like a charm.

Chapter 9.

FRUIT & WINE

Bananas, red or green apples, watermelon, dates, cantaloupe, pears, and grapes are the favorites of the SBB. These fruits satisfy the sugar cravings naturally and they don't create blood sugar spikes. SBBs make it a habit to eat two pieces of fruit a day, one in the morning and one in the evening.

Most fruits contain fiber, water and phytonutrients, so they work to feed the body and keep waste moving. Limit dried fruits to 3 pieces per serving.

OK, let's talk about wine for a minute. I'm not promoting drinking but if you do drink, studies have shown that red wine is good for the heart. I notice that SBBs don't drink a lot of hard liquor. Examples of hard liquors are whiskey, vodka, gin, etc. In other words, anything besides wine and beer.

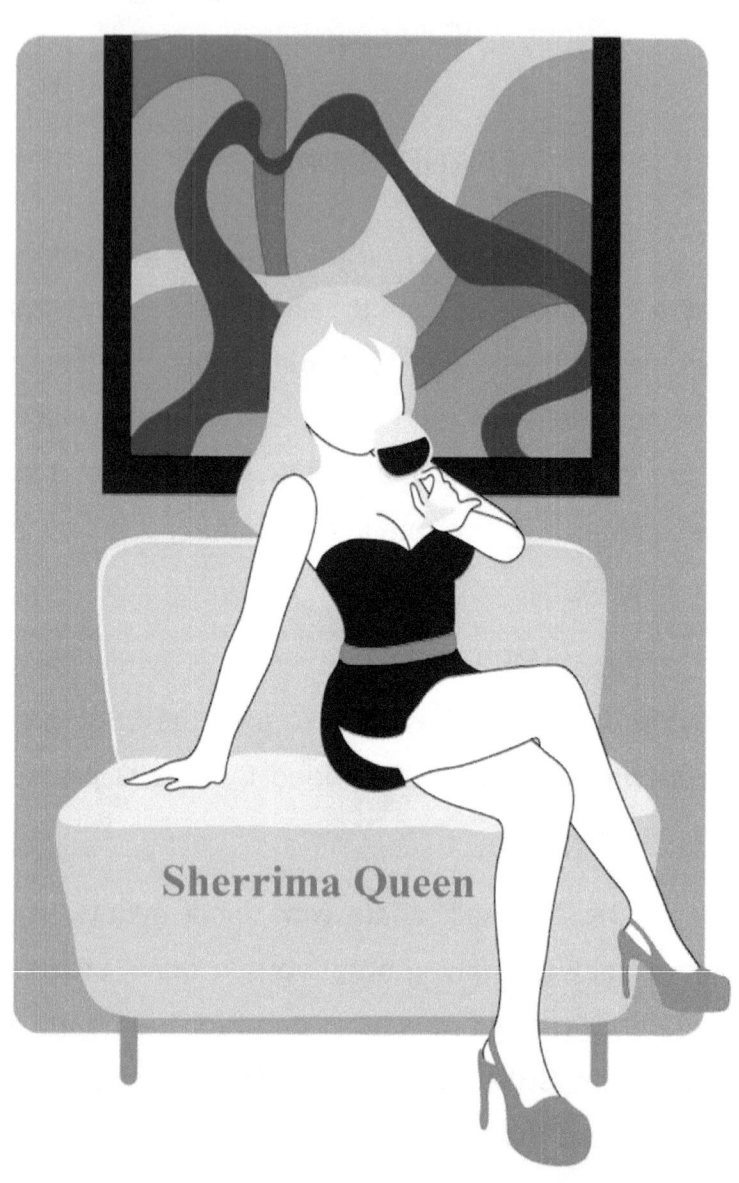

Sherrima Queen

Alcohol contains a lot of sugar because it's made from grains and it can contribute to weight gain. Also, too much can damage your liver. So instead SBBs drink wine, either white or red. Wine is made from grapes, which I'm sure you knew, and grapes contain resveratrol which is anti-aging. You probably won't be able to drink enough wine to achieve this benefit on its own, but as part of an overall diet that includes healthy plants like grapes, you'll see results.

Also, if you can find organic sulfite-free wine, that's even better. Sulfite is a chemical used as a preservative to prevent browning and discoloration in wine, mostly in white wine. Some people are allergic or have reactions to sulfites. However, Whole Foods sells sulfite-free wines and they're delicious. You can always do an after dinner drink like a cognac, which is also made from grapes, or a liquor made from nuts and herbs such as Frangelico. It's good to know that we have options.

If you love your white liquors below are some cocktails to consider. Try to stay away from fruit juices because of the sugar content. However, only drink once a week if you need to. The maximum is 2 drinks, period.

Cocktails that are OK to drink:

- ❖ Skinny girl margarita
- ❖ Vodka & tonic or club soda
- ❖ Gin & tonic or club soda
- ❖ Lite Beer

Chapter 10.

SEAFOOD: DON'T SHOOT THE MESSENGER

Seafood is a great alternative to red meat. A SBB eats seafood on occasion because it's a good source of protein, vitamins, minerals, and healthy fat. The most nutritious seafoods (omega 3 fatty acids) to eat are as follows: Wild caught salmon, wild Alaskan halibut, albacore tuna, and sardines.

Unfortunately, we even have to eat seafood in moderation if we eat it at all. Large amounts of mercury have been found in our seafood, particularly in larger fish such as salmon. The higher the fish is on the food chain, the more likely it is to contain mercury and PCBs (polychlorinated biphenyls). Mercury has been linked to cancer and levels in northern Pacific oceans have risen about 30 percent in the past 20 years, creating a concern for human consumption of seafood. PCBs are manufactured chemicals that have found their way from industry into our waterways and have been shown to have serious long-term effects on human and animal health.

Limit your intake of large fish to twice a week. Try to eat fish from deep-water ocean where fish are less likely to be contaminated, or eat smaller fish such as sardines. The chemicals that are being thrown in our oceans are hurting the sea life and us

I know you're probably asking, "I have to know where food comes from?" Yes, you do, especially if you care about your health. That's the world we live in. That's the main reason why we have to respect Mother Nature because she keeps us alive. Even with all her confidence a SBB needs Mother Earth.

Red Flags:

❖ Don't eat farm-raised fish. These fish are not fed a proper natural diet. They're given food that can contain chemicals.

❖ Always eat your seafood with lemon or

lime. It adds flavor, aids digestion and is filled with vitamin C. Once again, a SBB refrains from eating it fried but if you have to, remember - moderation!

❖ If fish smells "fishy" or looks slimy, it's past its prime. Don't buy it. It should have a somewhat dry look and a fresh smell, not a foul one.

❖ Beware of shellfish (crab, lobster, shrimp, oysters, mussels, clams). During some summer months, temperatures can be too hot and shellfish may become contaminated. The rule of thumb is, it's ok to eat shellfish in any month that has an "R" in it.

Chapter 11.

WHOLE GRAINS & CARBOHYDRATES

When a SBB thinks of Carbohydrates she thinks of whole grains because it's the only carbs she eats. Whole grains are a large group of organic compounds occurring in foods and living tissues, including sugars, starch and cellulose. Examples of carbs include rice, pasta, sweet potato and bread, to name a few. You want to eat most of your carbs before 7 p.m., especially on days that you work out. It will give you more energy and restore your muscles.

According to research, a person should eat 288 grams of carbs a day. Most vegetarians will eat more, because they don't eat meat and need the extra carbs to feel satisfied and give them energy. The healthiest whole grains to eat are quinoa or black rice, and they're also the most expensive. However, all the carbs listed below are considered good carbohydrates. A SBB wants anything and everything that's going to add value

44

to her body and keep her healthy. These grains listed below are the best on the market, thus far.

THE BEST GRAINS TO EAT

- ❖ Quinoa
- ❖ Black rice (find at Asian markets or high end supermarkets such as Publix or Whole Foods)
- ❖ Brown rice
- ❖ Whole wheat pasta
- ❖ Spelt
- ❖ Whole grain bread
- ❖ Ezekiel bread (made from sprouted grains and found in the frozen case)

It's important here to make the distinction between carbohydrates and complex carbohydrates. Fruit and veggies also contain carbohydrates - the complex kind, as for whole grain including rice and pasta.. Complex carbs have all their components intact and digest slowly so you don't get blood sugar spikes the way you would with processed carbs such as cakes, white flour products, candy, or pizza which have had most of their nutritional value removed.

Chapter 12.

MORE WAYS TO ENHANCE YOUR INNER SBB

If you stick to the plan, you'll see real results. Here are some more ways to help you speed up the process, stay hydrated, enhance your look, make things go more smoothly, boost your confidence, and maintain your focus on your goal.

DO DRINK THE WATER

All SBBs drink ten glasses of water a day. They are not basic bitches, that's why they take everything they do a step further. So why would they drink eight glasses of water like everyone else? If you really want to upgrade your H_2O game drink alkaline water. It has pH levels above 7, as opposed to regular tap water.

Tap water pH levels are lower than 6. Alkaline water can get a little pricey, so the next alternative would be spring water. Most people drink spring water anyway. If you can't afford spring water, filtered water is a great alternative. Water keeps the body hydrated. Also, as you begin to drop weight and lose fat, it gets rid of toxins that have been stored in the fat. This "flushing" in turn helps the weight drop faster.- H_2O keeps the skin glowing and the body fluid. Bottoms up with H_2O!

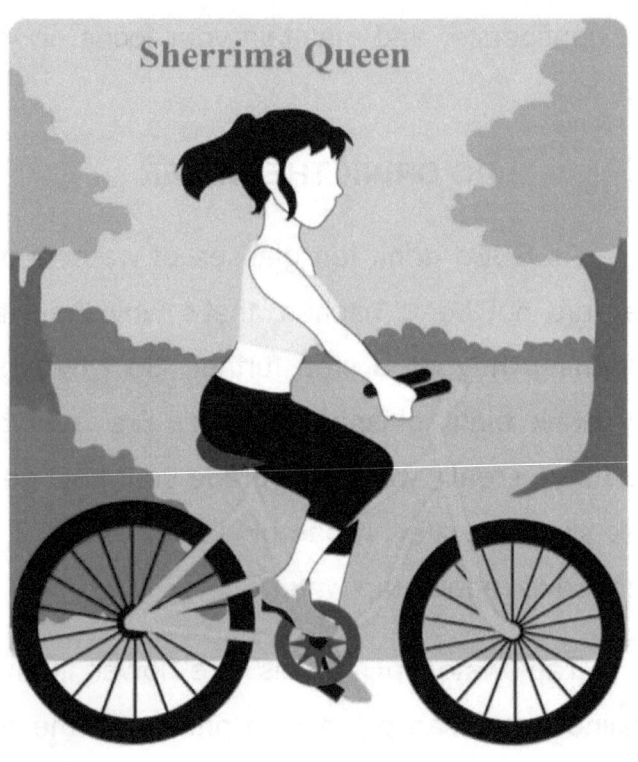

Sherrima Queen

SEX & EXERCISE

Every SBB knows the importance of exercise. That's why she works out a minimum of three times a week. She knows it's mandatory, even if she just goes for a walk. If you can do more, great!! Get that body moving.

When you exercise, you should do at least some form of cardio for a minimum of 30 minutes. The reason for this is to get all your internal organs and muscles warmed up and get your blood circulating to all the small capillaries that provide nourishment to the far corners of the body.

A treadmill, cycle or elliptical machine is awesome. In addition, buy yourself cute workout gear. It makes working out more fun and motivating when you know you look cute. Try to wear black leggings and bright colored tops. Believe me, this look will always have you on fleek when you're working out. Whoever wears it looks slimmer and sexy. Then take a picture for your Instagram.

You have to sweat! If you can't get to the gym, go for a jog around the neighborhood or park. It gets the job done. If you can't do that, have sex; at least you're getting your cardio in and it feel good. Even if it's a booty call. Just make sure you use protection. I'm not judging but don't loan him or her $100.

FAKE BITCH, DO YOU

If you have the money and want to go the plastic surgery route, go for it! SBBs make that appointment. I personally haven't had any plastic surgery, but there is nothing wrong with a nip here, a tuck there. Just make sure you don't go overboard and find yourself looking like a skinned cat with Ronald McDonald lips. You don't want your entire existence screaming fake! In addition, if you are considering plastic surgery, do your research and go to a reputable doctor.

Remember, a SBB is a leader, not a follower. She listens to her own heart, no matter what others think.

MEDITATION

A SBB meditates every day for at least 5 minutes minimum. If you can meditate longer, awesome. Get in quiet time with your mind. Whatever you can do is fine, morning or night, whatever works for you. If you can meditate every morning and night that would be awesome. If you don't know anything about meditation, take a class at your local Y.W.C.A. or online. Online classes have definitely enlightened me. There are also apps you can purchase that teach you about meditation. Meditation will calm your mind, allowing you to focus easier on your weight goals or other aspirations you have. When I meditate, I visualize the size I want to be and it gets me excited. Meditating helps you to reach your goals faster because you have universal energy supporting you. By the way, meditation has nothing to do with religion. It's good for the mind, body and soul.

CONFIDENCE

A SBB is confident about her body. She knows that her body is the vehicle that's being used to help her spirit grow. Therefore she knows her body is her temple and she treats it as such. She only puts food in it that will add value. A SBB is conscious about everything that goes into her mouth. A SBB develops the right mental attitude just like a boxer going into the ring. She is a winner and nothing can stop her. If you apply these changes to your diet and lifestyle, I know you will reach your goal. If you have moments of weakness, it's OK. Be patient with yourself. Every day is a new beginning, so try again tomorrow. This is what SBBs do. They never give up until they reach their goal. The new definition of a Bad Bitch is a Queen! Here's to all my Queens.

Chapter 13.

WHAT DO I DO NOW? THE 5-DAY MEAL PLAN

1. FOLLOW THE MEAL PLAN

2. MEDITATE EVERY DAY FOR 5 MINUTES OR MORE

3. DRINK 10 GLASSES OF WATER OR GREEN TEA A DAY

4. WORK OUT 3 TIMES A WEEK OR MORE

5. KEEP A POSITIVE ATTITUDE

YOU MOODY BITCH

After the first week of following the regimen in this book, you will have more energy, feel lighter and see yourself getting slimmer. On the flip side of that your personality may change. Some of you may become a moody bitch. You know in life you can't have a positive without a negative, but we're going to focus on the positive. The reason for the moodiness is because your body is purging old habits. It will be missing or craving your regular diet, sort of going through a withdrawal. Also, your cells are creating your new body. Fat cells will be shrinking. So, it might get a little challenging because there is a tug of war going on inside of you. Your body will want to return to your old ways, but please push through it. It will be worth it once you accomplish your goals.

I have listed a 5-day meal plan for you to follow and some suggested foods to get. You can substitute foods within the same group; it's up to you. However I do stress portion control. I do highly suggest sticking to the program in this book though if you want to see results faster. Once the weight starts falling off, which it will, you will be excited. Yay, you're becoming the person you were meant to be!

5 DAY MEAL PLAN

DAY 1: BREAKFAST

4 OUNCE CUP of hot oatmeal cereal or sugarless cold cereal (Bran flakes), with unsweetened organic almond, soy or low fat milk. You can also add fruit to your cereal as a natural sweetener.

Slice of whole grain toast with lite butter or honey

Green tea, orange juice or coffee

Or

20 oz. super fruit smoothie – Combine in a blender a handful of each

Frozen blueberries

Frozen strawberries

Kale

Banana

Your favorite protein mix (follow directions on the package)

2 ounces of almond milk, soy milk or water

DAY 1: LUNCH

Lean turkey breast with avocado on whole grain bread. If you're still hungry, add a small salad or soup.

Or

Kale, *bok choy or mixed green salad with grilled chicken and walnuts and a bowl of your favorite soup. If you're vegan, substitute tofu for chicken.

Don't forget to drink your 10 glasses of water throughout the day

DAY 1: MIDDAY SNACK (CHOOSE ONE)

½ or one small whole piece fresh fruit; for example, dates, apple, cantaloupe, watermelon. Pears are particularly high in fiber and watermelon is very hydrating.

Dry fruit (limit to 3 pieces)

Nuts such as almonds, walnuts, Brazil or cashew nuts. (limit to ¼ cup)

Tortilla chips (SBB loves Trader Joe's Veggie & Flaxseed flavor)

Carrot or celery sticks

DAY 1: DINNER

Broccoli soup

Small tossed green salad

Grilled halibut, steamed broccoli, brown rice or quinoa (vegans leave out fish and substitute sunflower seeds or slivered almonds sautéed in coconut oil)

DAY 1: DESSERT

Glass of red or white wine (no more than 4 ounces). You can add a few strawberries or other berries to your dessert.

Or

1" slice of flourless chocolate cake

Or

One small piece whole fruit

Try to limit your alcohol consumption to NO MORE THAN twice a week. Anything over that is not good for a SBB. Remember, you're trying to reach a goal.

*Bok Choy: Chinese vegetable that's rich in vitamins C and K. It has cancer-fighting properties for lung, colon and endometrial cancer.

DAY 2: BREAKFAST

Egg white omelette with spinach (2 eggs) or 2 hardboiled eggs and 1 slice of whole grain toast

1 piece of whole fruit

Coffee or green tea

Or

16 oz. super fruit smoothie (see recipe from Day 1)

DAY 2: LUNCH

Cup of tomato basil soup or favorite soup **(soups should be non-cream based)**

Grilled cheese sandwich (mozzarella or goat cheese) If vegan non dairy cheese, on whole grain bread

Or

Green salad with your choice of grilled chicken, tuna salad, Tofu, or lean beef one Slice of multigrain bread.

Two small slices of honeydew melon

If you need a snack, see the list from Day 1.

DAY 2: DINNER

Kale salad

Roasted chicken or your favorite fish; meat eaters can substitute 6 oz. of top sirloin steak; vegans substitute ¼ cup nuts or grilled tofu

Quinoa or any whole grain on the list

Dessert: Piece of pomegranate fruit

DAY 3: BREAKFAST

1 whole grain waffle with fruit and a tablespoon of pure maple syrup (do not use "pancake syrup")

4-6 ounces of grapefruit juice, coffee or green tea

DAY 3: LUNCH

Green salad with or without 4 ounces grilled or baked salmon (vegans substitute 4 ounces of Veggie protein for salmon)

Low or no sugar beverage such as unsweetened iced tea

Small red apple

DAY 3: DINNER

Steamed broccoli & carrots

Eggplant parmesan (use vegan cheese)

Or

7 oz. baked sliced turkey or lean beef with olive oil and red onion

Favorite steamed vegetable

2 oz. of quinoa

Day 3: Dessert: If needed

Choose one: One scoop of low fat ice cream; 1 cup baked apple slices with cinnamon and ginger; 1 ounce piece of dark chocolate

Or

4 ounce glass of wine

DAY 4: BREAKFAST

1 boiled egg or cereal

Coffee, green tea or orange juice

Or

20 oz. super fruit smoothie with protein mix

DAY 4: LUNCH

4-6 pieces of California or tuna sushi roll

Or

Bowl of vegetable soup with salad and 1 slice of whole grain bread

Or

4 ounce lean turkey burger

1 banana or another favorite fruit

Water with lemon (add a bit of honey if needed)

If you need a snack, choose one from day one snack list

DAY 4: DINNER

1 cup of pasta with sautéed onions and garlic; add 4 ounces favorite white or red meat

Or

3 oz. of black beans with brown rice

Bowl of butternut squash soup or favorite soup

Small salad

Or

Two vegan sausages (Tofurky makes a good one) or Italian sausage

Steamed veggies

DAY 4: DESSERT

None tonight

DAY 5: BREAKFAST

Super fruit smoothie with protein mix (your

favorite)

Coffee or tea

DAY 5: LUNCH

Spinach or Shanghai bok choy salad with 4 ounces of chicken or seafood with 10 almonds (or your favorite nuts)

Bowl of your favorite soup

Water, iced tea or low sugar beverage

Day 5: Snack

Non-GMO popcorn

Or

Favorite snack from day one

DAY 5: DINNER

2 small beef, fish or chicken tacos

Steamed red cabbage & asparagus mixed

Glass of low sugar beverage or 4 ounces wine since it's Friday

DAY 5: DESSERT

Another glass of wine or small slice of your favorite dessert

Other foods that are great to eat for weight loss:

1. Chickpeas

2. Artichoke hearts

3. Baked sweet potatoes

4. Green beans

5. Scallions

6. Black beans

7. Mushrooms

8. Wild rice

9. Squash

10. Tofu

11. Brussels sprouts

12. Tomatoes

13. Turkey burger

14. Salmon burger

This is an example of a typical SBB diet for 5 days. You may substitute any of the foods to your liking, but I suggest you follow the course outlined. As a general guideline, remember that your goal in eating is to eliminate high fat, high sugar and highly processed foods. Add more fresh fruits and veggies, lean meats and fish, water, green tea, and organically raised and grown products. Also, stay away from artificial sweeteners. When I say low sugar, I don't mean diet drinks, I mean water or tea with a bit of honey.

This book is meant as a beginner guide to start you off on your journey, so it only covers five days. On the sixth day, repeat the plan from one of the five days meal plans, whatever one is your favorite.

The seventh day is your chill day, so eat what you like. You can find recipes online, but remember it's about portion control. Just remember that you're a SBB and you practice self-control, so be particular about what and how much you put into your mouth.

If you substitute any foods, keep a food journal. It helps you to remember what you ate and how much. All the major diet plans recommend this and so do I, so I have left a few blank pages in the back of this book for that purpose.

Stay Healthy!

I love you all and good luck on your lifestyle journey!

www.ingramcontent.com/pod-product-compliance
Lightning Source LLC
Chambersburg PA
CBHW022345290526
45786CB00014B/2503